Dash Diet

Exquisite And Convenient Recipes: Ignite Your Path To
Health And Enhance Your Vitality: Uncover Efficient
Approaches And Enduring Outcomes

*(The Definitive Compendium Of Delectable Recipes For
Reducing Blood Pressure)*

SHAUN LANGEVIN

TABLE OF CONTENT

What Is The Definition Or Concept Of The Dash Diet?

When considering the comprehensive understanding of the DASH Diet, it is imperative to contemplate a few fundamental facets. As you may be aware, the dietary choices we make have a profound impact on our holistic health. Consequently, a diet containing detrimental components such as cholesterol and saturated fats clearly contributes to the development of hypertension and a multitude of other detrimental illnesses. Nevertheless, the consumption of appropriate dietary choices can mitigate the likelihood of experiencing such detrimental health conditions. There exists a specialized dietary regimen that has been formulated with the aim of reducing elevated blood pressure levels, commonly referred to as hypertension. This specific dietary regimen is known as the DASH Diet.

What is the essence of this matter?" or "What is the purpose of this inquiry?

The NHBL institute's clinical studies indicate a recommendation for the adoption of the DASH Diet. Following meticulous analysis and comprehensive clinical trials, the scientific community has arrived at the determination that adhering to a dietary regimen abundant in magnesium, potassium, calcium, fiber, and protein has the capacity to markedly reduce elevated blood pressure levels. Moreover, the research substantiated the notion that adhering to a diet rich in fruits and vegetables while minimizing fat intake can significantly diminish the likelihood of developing hypertension. Additionally, the diet exhibits prompt efficacy, requiring minimal time to manifest the desired outcomes.

The DASH diet places its primary emphasis on three key components: magnesium, potassium, and calcium.

These nutrients have been identified for their capacity to mitigate elevated blood pressure levels. According to a study report, a typical 2000 calorie diet contains approximately 500 milligrams of magnesium, 1.2 grams of calcium, and 4.7 grams of potassium.

Using the DASH Diet

Implementing and adhering to a DASH diet is rather uncomplicated and clear-cut, as it requires minimal effort in meal preparation. In addition to the avoidance of high-cholesterol foods, the dieter is also encouraged to increase the incorporation of vegetables, cereals, and fruits to the greatest extent feasible. In light of the fact that the foods incorporated into the DASH diet are abundant in fiber, it is highly recommended that individuals gradually increase their consumption of fiber-rich foods to prevent potential gastrointestinal issues and diarrhea. Furthermore, you can enhance your dietary fiber intake by incorporating an additional portion of fruits and vegetables into your daily nutrition.

Grains, along with B vitamins and minerals, serve as valuable sources of dietary fiber. As an example, various additional grain products such as whole grains, bran, wheat breads, wheat germ, and low fat cereals can be employed to augment one's dietary fiber intake.

Conduct a thorough examination of the ingredient listings on packaged and processed food items. Select food items that are characterized by lower levels of cholesterol, saturated fats, sodium, chocolates, and similar substances. If one intends to consume meat, it is advisable to restrict their daily consumption to a maximum of six ounces. Additionally, skim milk or low-fat milk can serve as alternative sources of protein.

The DASH diet is gaining significant traction among individuals who prioritize their health, primarily due to its lack of necessity for elaborate recipes or specialized meals. There are no specific limitations with regards to calorie monitoring and cooking methods, provided that one refrains from consuming foods that are high in cholesterol and saturated fats. The DASH diet regimen is a nutritionally balanced eating plan that focuses on three vital minerals, known to have a favorable impact on hypertension.

The Plan For Promoting Wellness And Vitality

The DASH diet entails the prioritization of portion regulation through the consumption of a diverse range of foods, ensuring the attainment of adequate nutritional content from each of the essential food groups. By adhering to the program, it is possible to achieve a reduction in blood pressure within a span of two weeks, with the potential to see a decrease of up to fourteen points within the duration of eight weeks.

The Sodium Levels

In addition to providing a variety of choices centered around fruits, vegetables, and low-dairy foods, the standard diet plan also entails a reduced intake of whole grains. The conventional dietary regimen permits a daily intake of 2,300 milligrams (mg). In contrast, the reduced sodium variation of the dash diet regimen imposes a daily limit of just 1,500 mg.

In addition to their merits, both variations of the DASH alternative yield a substantial reduction in sodium consumption as compared to typical American diets, potentially mitigating an excessive influx of up to 3,400 mg of sodium per day.

Based on the guidelines established by the American Heart Association, it is recommended that adults restrict their daily sodium intake to a maximum of 1,500 mg. It is recommended to consult with your healthcare provider to ensure that you are consuming quantities that fall within your prescribed limits. Various elements are taken into account, encompassing your ethnicity, age, and pre-existing or present medical conditions.

Address the issue of excessive salt consumption by eliminating the presence of salt shakers on the dinner table. During the process of preparing meals, opt for condiments and foods that are either sodium-free or low in sodium. It is imperative to refrain from consuming foods that have undergone the process of pickling, smoking, or curing.

The Influence of Alcohol

The supervision of alcohol consumption should be diligently undertaken. It is recommended that women limit their alcohol intake to no more than one drink per day, while men are advised to consume a maximum of two drinks within a 24-hour period. In addition to mitigating the risk of developing high blood pressure, you are also aiding in the pursuit of weight management. Furthermore, excessive consumption of alcohol can lead to a sudden increase in blood pressure.

Within a span of two weeks since the initiation of the DASH Diet regimen, empirical evidence has demonstrated a notable reduction in blood pressure levels. The elemental constituents pivotal to this composition are magnesium, calcium, and potassium. In conclusion, the DASH diet regimen effectively restricts sodium and salt consumption, while alternative approaches may offer comparatively lesser reductions. Excessive sodium consumption can lead to fluid retention, thereby elevating pressure and exertion on the cardiac system, ultimately resulting in an increase in blood pressure.

Cancer Prevention
The substantial presence of antioxidants, vitamins, and fiber confers advantages for specific types of cancer. Vegetables, whole grains, and fruits are rich sources of these vital nutrients. These dietary items assist in mitigating the repercussions of the waste substances generated during cellular respiration, which possess the potential to induce aberrant cellular growth, subsequently fostering the proliferation of cancerous cells.

Lowered Cholesterol

As one ingests the entire grain, they are supplying their body with a natural fiber source derived from oats, brown rice, and comparable items. Through the intake of an adequate amount of fiber, as documented by scientific research, you will effectively lower your cholesterol levels.

The recommended daily intake of dietary fiber for women is approximately 25 grams, while men are advised to consume around 38 grams on a daily basis.

Avoid Diabetes
By abstaining from starchy foods and devoid of empty carbohydrates, you can effectively evade the ingestion of "simple" sugars that are promptly assimilated by your body and swiftly transported into your bloodstream. This consumption can lead to a spike in insulin levels and an increase in the body's glucose levels, thereby elevating the risk of developing diabetes.

Kidney Health

Efforts can be made to mitigate the occurrence of kidney stones, a condition that may lead to severe discomfort. The dietary regimen inhibits the formation of mineral deposits responsible for the genesis of calculi. The excessive intake of sodium can result in renal insufficiency as well. DASH has garnered acclaim from the esteemed National Kidney Foundation for its inherent potential in benefiting individuals who may be susceptible to kidney failure. Once more, it is advisable to engage in a conversation regarding this matter with your healthcare professional.

Osteoporosis

The DASH program comprises a significant concentration of potassium, protein, and calcium, thereby aiding in the deceleration of the progression or commencement of osteoporosis.

The meal consists of a combination of low-fat proteins, green vegetables, dairy products, whole grains, and fruits, thereby facilitating the development of strong skeletal structure.

Weight Issues

You will acquire the skills necessary to prioritize crucial factors that contribute to improved nutrition and increased physical activity. The outcomes will become evident upon devising a strategy and diligently adhering to it.

In order to achieve weight loss, it is necessary to attain a state of calorie deficit. The DASH diet promotes the consumption of nutrient-dense foods instead of calorie-rich foods, which can effectively aid in significant weight loss. The inclusion of ample fiber content, along with a selection abundant in essential nutrients, further enhances the appeal of this dietary regimen.

Pose yourself these supplementary inquiries:

• What objectives do you have in mind to achieve while following the DASH Diet Plan?

Could you kindly indicate your optimal weight for good health?

• What are the potential health risks associated with BMI, and what impact do they have on an individual?

The Solution for Optimal Weight Management

Accelerate the Rate

• It is advised to restrict the consumption of beverages containing high amounts of sugar, confectioneries, red meat, and sodium.

• Increase consumption of fruits, low-fat dairy products, and vegetables.

• Increase consumption of nuts, poultry, fish, and whole-grain foods.

• Significantly reduce consumption of foods containing elevated levels of trans fats, saturated fats, and cholesterol.

Make Gradual Changes

Please refrain from hastening your actions; occasionally, a more moderate pace yields superior results. Commence by restricting sodium intake to a maximum of one teaspoon or 2,400 milligrams on a daily basis. Once you have accustomed yourself to that quantity, endeavor to reduce it to 2/3 teaspoons or 1,500 milligrams per day. That sum should encompass food items that are consumed, as well as any additional components added during the meal.

Understanding Dash Diet

Instead of viewing the DASH diet as a mere dietary plan, it should be regarded as a transformative and sustainable shift in one's lifestyle. The National Institutes of Health (NIH) has devised this program to cater to individuals diagnosed with hypertension, granting them the opportunity to savor their preferred culinary choices, while simultaneously striving towards the reduction or normalization of their blood pressure levels. With the purpose of offering a diverse, delicious, and nutritionally-sound menu, the diet incorporates nourishing food choices and employs healthier cooking methods to prepare favored meals.

This dietary plan does not aim specifically for weight reduction.

Instead, it emphasizes a novel perspective on food consumption, prioritizing health over weight loss.

While the primary purpose of the DASH diet does not encompass weight loss, it is frequently observed that individuals tend to shed pounds as a consequence of adhering to this dietary regimen. Individuals who have elevated blood pressure or are predisposed to it can significantly reap the advantages of weight loss. Obesity represents a prominent determinant of elevated blood pressure, while concurrently augmenting the risk of various afflictions commonly associated with high blood pressure, including but not limited to stroke and cardiovascular ailments, specifically among individuals with a body mass index (BMI) of 30 or higher.

Strategies for Reducing Sodium Intake

The DASH diet presents recommendations pertaining to both sodium consumption and caloric intake. Both the standard DASH diet as well as its low-sodium variant permit a maximum intake of 2,300 milligrams (mg) of sodium per day. In contrast to the typical dietary habits of the average American, wherein an intake of 3,500 mg of sodium per day is observed, the amount included herein is notably lower.

Augment your dietary fiber intake

The DASH diet advocates the consumption of a higher amount of dietary fiber than one would typically consume. High-fiber vegetables, fruits, and grains constitute a vital component of this dietary regimen as they not only contribute to the reduction of blood pressure but also provide satiety and lasting satisfaction throughout the day.

Furthermore, the diet's elevated fiber content contributes to weight loss efforts through its ability to maintain stable blood sugar levels within safe parameters.

Place a Focus on Beneficial Fats

A key component of the DASH diet is to incorporate ample amounts of nutritious fats while moderating the intake of detrimental fats. In an effort to decrease the intake of saturated and trans fats in the diet, processed and fast foods are replaced by unprocessed, nutrient-dense foods such as low-fat dairy products, lean meats, omega-3–rich fish, seafood, nuts, and seeds.

Through the reduction of LDL cholesterol and the elevation of HDL cholesterol, these more nutritious fat alternatives enhance the overall well-being of individuals. Cardiovascular disease is perilous and among the prominent hazards linked to elevated blood pressure, thus this holds particular significance for individuals afflicted by the latter.

Minimize your intake of alcoholic beverages and caffeinated substances.

While the consumption of these beverages is not explicitly prohibited, it is advisable to exercise moderation due to their limited nutritional content, potential to elevate blood pressure, and frequent inclusion of substantial amounts of sugar. The DASH diet advises restricting the consumption of sugary foods to a maximum of five servings per day, citing the association between elevated blood pressure and the occurrence of metabolic syndrome and type 2 diabetes. If one takes pleasure in savoring a glass of wine during mealtime or indulging in an intermittent cocktail, there is no need for despair as these indulgences can still be relished in moderation.

This also applies to your morning coffee, your afternoon tea, or your preferred afternoon soft drink. One can derive pleasure from these beverages, provided that they adhere to the remaining dietary and physical activity recommendations and consume them in accordance with the prescribed minimal and health-conscious dosage.

An Optimal Ingestion of Essential Nutrients

The comprehensive range of fruits, vegetables, grains, and other whole foods embedded in the DASH diet guarantees the adequate intake of essential vitamins and minerals necessary for maintaining optimal health. Nevertheless, it additionally furnishes a wholesome abundance of minerals recognized for their capacity to enhance or diminish blood pressure, for instance magnesium and potassium. Adequate quantities of these minerals can be obtained through the consumption of ample servings of green vegetables, bananas, and legumes.

"Individual customization is available for your caloric and sodium intake.

According to the guidelines of the standard DASH diet, an individual may consume a maximum of 2,300 mg of sodium per day, whereas the reduced sodium DASH diet permits a maximum intake of 1,500 mg of sodium per day. Alternatively, you have the option to consume a diet that supplies a daily caloric range of 1,500-3,100 calories. The selection and combination of calorie and sodium limits will variably rely upon your individual requirements.

You have the option, in consultation with your healthcare provider, to opt for a reduced calorie diet if you are carrying excess weight, or a higher calorie diet if you lead an highly active lifestyle or simply wish to sustain your present weight. If you do not currently have high blood pressure but wish to prevent its occurrence in the future, you have the option to opt for an increased sodium intake. If you currently experience high blood pressure or are at a significant risk of developing it due to factors such as being overweight or having a family history of the condition, it is advisable to opt for the sodium level that is comparatively lower.

The various sodium and calorie plans can be integrated in whichever manner is most suitable for your present state of well-being and your objectives.

The History

In 1992, the National Institutes of Health (NIH) provided funding for a study aimed at addressing the escalating prevalence of hypertension in the United States through dietary interventions. The objective was to develop a dietary regimen capable of mitigating or enhancing hypertension. The National Heart, Lung, and Blood Institute (NHLBI), a subsidiary of the National Institutes of Health (NIH), undertook this research endeavor in collaboration with esteemed and pioneering medical research establishments across the United States. The aforementioned institutions comprised Johns Hopkins University, Brigham and Women's Hospital, Kaiser Permanente Center for Health Research, Duke University Medical Center, and Pennington Biomedical Research Center.

The aforementioned five institutions, in conjunction with the NHLBI, have conducted the most comprehensive research on hypertension ever undertaken within our nation's borders. The data amassed by this consortium of scholars throughout an extended duration culminated in the development of the Dietary Approaches to Stop Hypertension diet, recognized as the DASH diet.

The DASH diet has subsequently gained widespread recognition as being one of the most healthful dietary regimens to adhere to. In the year 2012, the revised Dietary Guidelines for Americans advocated for the adoption of the DASH diet by individuals of all age groups, encompassing children and older adults, irrespective of the presence or absence of hypertension. Indeed, the newly introduced MyPlate dietary guidelines, which have replaced the previous food pyramid, are predominantly founded upon the principles of the DASH diet guidelines.

The Scientific Rationale Underlying the Dash Diet

Throughout the duration of the investigation pertaining to the issues relating to hypertension and the potential ameliorating effects of nutrition, multiple cohorts composed of medical practitioners, nurses, and statisticians collaborated with the respective institutions, undertaking a multitude of clinical trials at each of the facilities. The research involved the screening of over eight thousand American individuals, with approximately two-thirds of them belonging to high-risk groups including but not limited to African Americans, individuals with family histories of high blood pressure, and those who were overweight. The individuals participating in the study were provided with three distinct dietary interventions.

The Dietary Regimens That Precipitated The Development Of The Dash Diet

The initial dietary regimen, which closely resembled the conventional American diet, was deemed as the control factor. The sole distinction observed between this eating regimen and the customary American diet was the comparatively reduced consumption of sodium, amounting to 1,500 milligrams on a daily basis. The objective of this dietary intervention was to evaluate the impact of the reduced sodium regimen typically advised by physicians for individuals diagnosed with hypertension.

The second dietary regimen incorporated a reduced quantity of between-meal snacks and an increased proportion of fruits and vegetables in comparison to the customary American diet. The fiber content in the meal was considerably greater compared to the typical daily dietary intake of the average American. The objective of this dietary regimen was to examine the effects of a high-fiber nutritional plan on individuals with elevated blood pressure.

The third dietary plan is the one that eventually evolved into the DASH diet. Similarly to the second dietary plan, it consisted primarily of fiber-rich foods, fruits, and vegetables. Furthermore, the product exhibited a notably reduced quantity of saturated fats while boasting elevated levels of essential minerals such as potassium and magnesium, widely recognized for their potential to ameliorate hypertension. Nevertheless, the prescribed sodium consumption on this dietary regimen amounted to 3,000 milligrams per diem. The significant presence of sodium can be attributed to the researchers' objective of investigating the potential benefits of implementing dietary modifications beyond sodium reduction in mitigating high blood pressure.

Comprehensive Investigation, Promising Findings

These diets were employed in two distinct trials. In both experiments, every group was subjected to the initial diet for a period of three weeks, during which their blood pressure, symptoms, and urine were closely monitored. After a duration of three weeks, a total of four hundred participants were chosen to proceed with the trial, whereby they would be assigned to one of the three dietary interventions.

The data obtained from the initial trial indicated that the implementation of a low-sodium control diet resulted in a demonstrated reduction in the participants' blood pressure levels. The DASH diet also provided some assistance, albeit not to a satisfactory extent. In the subsequent trial, modifications were made to the DASH diet regimen to incorporate reduced sodium consumption.

By the end of the second study, it was observed that the control diet continued to exhibit a positive impact on blood pressure. However, the newly introduced DASH diet yielded significantly more favorable outcomes, leading to a considerably greater reduction in blood pressure.

Indeed, it has been discovered by researchers that following the new DASH diet for a mere thirty days yielded a significant decrease in blood pressure. Specifically, individuals identified as being prone to high blood pressure experienced an average reduction of 8.9/4.5 mm Hg (systolic/diastolic), while those already diagnosed with hypertension exhibited an average decrease of 11.5/5.7 mm Hg.

Furthermore, it was revealed by researchers that the newly devised DASH diet not only resulted in a reduction of harmful cholesterol levels, but also effectively decreased overall body fat, primarily targeting perilous abdominal fat deposits. Scientists attribute these advantages to the decreased consumption of sugar, as the reduction of sugar intake enhances insulin sensitivity and facilitates the process of fat reduction.

As a consequence of the research findings, the DASH diet has emerged as a widely endorsed dietary regimen, particularly for individuals with heightened concerns pertaining to hypertension.

Almond And Apricot Biscotti

Ingredients

- 2 tablespoons canola oil
- 2 tablespoons dark honey
- 1/2 teaspoon almond extract
- 2/3 cup chopped dried apricots
- 1/4 cup coarsely chopped almonds
- 3/4 cup whole-wheat (whole-meal) flour
- 3/4 cup all-purpose (plain) flour
- 1/4 cup firmly packed brown sugar
- 1 teaspoon baking powder
- 2 eggs, lightly beaten
- 2 tablespoons 1 percent low-fat milk

Directions

Set the oven temperature to 350 degrees Fahrenheit in preparation.

Using a sizable mixing bowl, blend together the flours, brown sugar, and baking powder. Whisk to blend. Incorporate the eggs, milk, canola oil, honey, and almond extract into the mixture. Agitate the ingredients using a wooden utensil until the dough reaches the initial stages of cohesion. Add the chopped apricots and almonds. Using hands dusted with flour, thoroughly combine the ingredients until the dough is fully incorporated.

Position the dough upon a lengthy piece of plastic wrap and manually sculpt it into a compressed log measuring 12 inches in length, 3 inches in width, and approximately 1 inch in height. Carefully remove the plastic wrap and transfer the dough onto a baking sheet that has been coated with a nonstick surface. Bake until a pale golden color is achieved, approximately 25 to 30 minutes. Relocate the contents onto a separate baking sheet to allow for a cooling period of 10 minutes. Please ensure that the oven remains at a temperature of 350 degrees Fahrenheit.

Position the appropriately cooled log onto the surface of a cutting board. Using a serrated knife, make diagonal cuts to create 24 slices that are 1/2 inch wide, running in a crosswise direction. Organize the slices in a downward-facing position on the baking sheet. Proceed to place it back in the oven and continue baking until it becomes crispy, for a duration of 15 to 20 minutes. Relocate the baked goods onto a wire rack and allow them to cool thoroughly. Place in a tightly sealed receptacle.

Pumpkin Smoothie For Morning Nourishment

Ingredients:

- 1/2 cup vanilla yogurt
- 3 teaspoons cinnamon
- Graham crackers, crushed (cinnamon-flavored)
- 1 can froze pumpkin pie filling (8-ounce)
- 1 1/2 cup whole milk

Directions:

Incorporate the yogurt and one cup of milk within the blender.

Incorporate the frozen pumpkin pie filling and pulse until thorough integration of the ingredients is achieved.

Incorporate the remaining 1/2 cups of milk into the mixture until thoroughly blended.

Present in a generously sized glass, garnished with fragments of cinnamon-infused graham crackers.

Serve right away.

Walnut-Cranberry Oatmeal

Ingredients:

- 4 teaspoons of walnuts, chopped
- 2 cups of water
- ¼ of a teaspoon of ground cinnamon
- 1 cup of steel cut oats
- ¼ teaspoon of salt
- 1/3 of a cup of dried cranberries
- 4 teaspoons of brown sugar

Directions:

Incorporate the steel oats, cranberries, salt, cinnamon, and water within a saucepan. Proceed to rapidly heat the mixture until it reaches boiling point, then promptly lower the heat and maintain a gentle simmer for a duration of 20 minutes, until a desired creamy consistency is achieved. Divide the mixture equally among four bowls. Include a single teaspoon of brown sugar and walnuts into every individual bowl.

Additionally, it is possible to replace the walnuts with any fruit of your preference.

Southwestern Potato Skins

Ingredients:

6 slices turkey bacon, cooked until crisp, chopped

1 medium tomato, diced

2 tablespoons sliced green onions

1/2 cup shredded cheddar cheese

6 large baking potatoes

1 teaspoon olive oil

1 teaspoon chili powder

1/8 teaspoon Tabasco sauce

Directions:

Kindly set the oven temperature to 450 degrees Fahrenheit prior to use. Apply a thin layer of cooking spray to the baking sheet.

Thoroughly cleanse the potatoes and puncture each one multiple times using a fork. Heat the uncovered microwave on high setting until the food reaches a tender consistency, which usually takes approximately 10 minutes. Take out the potatoes from the microwave and transfer them onto a wire rack to allow for adequate cooling. Once the potatoes have cooled sufficiently, slice them in half longitudinally and carefully remove the inner flesh, ensuring that a layer approximately 1/4 inch thick remains attached to the skin.

In a compact bowl, blend the olive oil, chili powder, and hot sauce using a whisk. Apply the olive oil mixture onto the interior of the potato skins. Divide each half of the potato skin further into quarters by cutting them crosswise. Arrange the potatoes onto the baking sheet.

In a compact container, delicately combine the turkey bacon, tomato, and onions. Stuff each potato skin with the aforementioned mixture and proceed to garnish with a layer of cheese.

* Continue baking until the cheese has thoroughly melted and the potato skins have been fully heated, approximately 10 minutes. Serve immediately.

Tomato Bruschetta

Ingredients:

1/2 cup diced fennel

1 teaspoon olive oil

2 teaspoons balsamic vinegar

1 teaspoon black pepper

1/2 whole-grain baguette, cut into six 1/2-inch-thick diagonal slices

2 tablespoons chopped basil

1 tablespoon chopped parsley

2 cloves garlic, minced

3 tomatoes, diced

Directions:

Proceed toasting the baguette slices in a preheated oven set at 400 degrees

Fahrenheit, until they achieve a slight golden-brown color.

* Combine all remaining ingredients in a compact bowl.

Distribute the mixture uniformly onto the toasted bread. Serve immediately.

Pineapple Oat Breakfast

Ingredients:

- 1 cup walnuts, chopped
- 2 fresh fresh eggs
- 1 tbsp. stevia
- 2 tsp. vanilla extract

- 2 cups pineapple, cubed
- 1 tbsp ginger, grated
- 2 cups skim milk
- 2 cups oats, old-fashioned

Kindly ensure that the oven is preheated to a temperature of 400 degrees Fahrenheit.

Combine the oats, pineapple, walnuts, and ginger in a generously sized bowl, ensuring they are mixed together evenly. Agitate the mixture and carefully transfer it to a baking pan that has been coated with a thin layer of cooking spray.

In a moderately large bowl, diligently blend together the milk, eggs, stevia, and vanilla.

Pour the mixture onto the oats.

Place in the oven and cook for a duration of 25 minutes, or until fully cooked and firm.

Serve warm.

Does The Dash Diet Live Up To Its Reputation?

One of the primary objectives of the DASH diet, among various other components, is to provide instruction and guidance to individuals suffering from hypertension, in order to promote a dietary regimen that effectively mitigates the detrimental consequences associated with elevated blood pressure levels. By adhering to the principles of the DASH diet, it is plausible to surmise that the likelihood of developing heart diseases, stroke, and kidney stones may be diminished to a manageable extent.

Advantages of the DASH Diet "

Several scholarly studies have demonstrated that adherence to the DASH diet recommendations enables individuals with hypertension to effectively manage their blood pressure levels. Hypertension is a leading contributor to global mortality. In addition, hypertension is also a contributing factor to elevated rates of diabetes, cardiovascular ailments, and osteoporosis.

These illnesses pose a significant challenge in terms of treatment due to their chronic nature. Due to the exorbitant cost of medication, some individuals may find it unfeasible to pursue treatment, which is why the DASH diet emphasizes preventative measures as an alternative.

Elevated levels of cholesterol in the bloodstream can have detrimental effects on human well-being. This is because it leads to the thickening of blood vessels, thereby posing a substantial threat to human life.

The DASH diet includes food options that are low in cholesterol, or entirely devoid of it. The inclusion of food items such as fruits, low-fat dairy products, and vegetables in the DASH diet has been shown to effectively reduce the risk of developing hypertension over an extended period of time.

A number of foods incorporated in the DASH diet possess the capacity to mitigate the sodium levels within the body.

Numerous health professionals propose that, under typical conditions, a well-functioning human organism necessitates a daily intake of 2400 mg of sodium. In contrast to conventional cuisine, this level of sodium content has the potential to escalate to 3500 mg, a quantity deemed detrimental particularly in terms of blood pressure regulation.

Elevated sodium concentrations can contribute to the escalation of blood pressure, subsequently leading to the development of hypertension. If left unaddressed, this condition may ultimately result in fatality.

In addition to remedying hypertension, the DASH diet includes a substantial amount of dietary fiber, which effectively supports optimal digestive functioning within the gastric system. Efficient digestion results in the complete absorption of essential nutrients into the body, leading to optimal energy levels and enhanced fat metabolism.

When there is a decrease in the accumulated adipose tissue, there is a greater probability that the individual will experience long-term weight reduction. Henceforth, the DASH diet represents the superior choice when contrasted with the conventional diet.

Ultimately, individuals who typically express symptoms related to inflammation within their bodily tissues, particularly the cardiac region, experience positive outcomes from adopting the DASH diet. The DASH diet is characterized by reduced levels of cholesterol. Elevated cholesterol levels contribute to the narrowing of blood vessels, consequently impeding the efficient delivery of oxygen-rich blood to various areas of the body. An individual afflicted with vascular thickening commonly exhibits fatigue as a result of compromised oxygenation throughout the body. The DASH diet is specifically endorsed for individuals diagnosed with hypertension, thus promoting an extension of their lifespan.

Integration Of The Dash Diet Into Your Daily Routine

Given that we have thoroughly explored the DASH diet and its prominent advantages, it is only reasonable to aspire to commence adhering to this dietary regimen promptly. However, a crucial inquiry that must be posed is: What strategies can be employed to seamlessly integrate the DASH diet into one's daily routine?

Considering the prevalence of elevated sodium levels in restaurant meals and pre-packaged foods, how can one effectively integrate a dietary regimen into their daily life, while simultaneously savoring favored culinary choices and indulging in dining experiences at cherished establishments alongside loved ones?

To commence, it is advisable to incorporate a greater quantity of fruits and vegetables into one's daily dietary intake. Therefore, it is recommended to opt for dishes that incorporate fruits or incorporate greens, as they are highly recommended food choices within the prescribed diet. It is imperative to eliminate from one's diet foods that possess elevated levels of saturated fats, cholesterol, and trans fats. While this may not be optimal while on the move, it can be easily accomplished at home by selecting food items that are low in these indicators, which are known to contribute to hypertension and elevated blood pressure levels.

It is advisable to restrict the consumption of red meat. Therefore, a simple approach to achieve this objective would be to opt for alternative sources of low-fat proteins throughout the course of the day. One may opt for consuming poultry, alternative sources of meat and seafood, or consider the inclusion of protein shakes as part of their dietary regimen. There is no requirement for you to completely eliminate red meat; instead, it is advisable to restrict its consumption.

A convenient snack option would be nuts, which are rich in essential healthy fats and can be easily transported to various locations. If one is in a state of hunger and requires a swift refreshment, they can be conveniently obtained. Moreover, it is imperative to refrain from consuming processed foods. Thus, opting for whole grains is recommended over white bread.

If you are seeking uncomplicated recipe suggestions and aim to seamlessly integrate the dietary regimen into your way of life, there is an abundance of ideas available to explore. You are merely restricting the consumption of processed foods, confections, and refined sugars, instead opting for alternatives that consist solely of natural ingredients. The quantity of sodium consumed may vary from day to day, which is acceptable. The objective of the dietary plan is to help you maintain a proximity to the suggested mean value over a specified duration. Furthermore, given the abundance of food manufacturers offering low sodium alternatives, it is highly attainable to adhere to the recommended daily limit or come remarkably close to it throughout the entirety of the week.

The DASH Diet is surprisingly uncomplicated to adhere to, and does not entail significant alterations to successfully incorporate it into your daily routine. You are effectively restricting your sodium consumption, eliminating refined and processed foods, and opting for all-natural alternatives (i.e. - consuming the appropriate foods). It imposes no significant restrictions on the types of food you can consume, except for regulating portion sizes, while offering guidelines for making more health-conscious choices. As a result, it proves to be one of the more seamless dietary transitions and easily sustainable on a daily basis.

Whole-Grain Pancakes

Ingredients:

- 1/4 cup rolled oats
- 3 tbsp honey
- 1 tbs oil
- 2 1/4 cups soy milk
- 3 large egg whites
- 1 cup whole-wheat flour
- 1/4 cup millet flour
- 1/2 cup barley flour
- 1 1/2 tbsp baking powder
- 2 tbsp flaxseed (ground)

Directions:

Incorporate the millet flour, whole-wheat flour, barley flour, baking powder, flaxseed, and rolled oats within a spacious bowl.

In a separate bowl, combine the soy milk, honey, egg whites, and oil using a whisk and proceed to pour this mixture onto the dry ingredients. Mix until just blended. Allow the batter to rest for approximately 30 minutes within the confines of the refrigerator.

Carefully apply a thin layer of oil to a skillet and place it on the stove over medium heat. Using a measuring cup, dispense approximately 1/4 cup of batter into the skillet. Proceed to cook until the batter has solidified and there is a browned outer rim. Rotate the item to achieve browning on the opposite side. Continue this process until all of the batter has been used. Garnish the heated pancake with a generous dusting of cinnamon sugar or elevate its taste with the addition of freshly sliced fruits before savoring it.

Double-Boiled White Beans In The Porto Style

Ingredients:

1 clove of garlic pounded

Salt

Black pepper

Red pepper

Oil

2 tomatoes

500 gram of double white bean

3 cups of cooked white beans

2 clubs

1 small onion, finely chopped

Chive

Preparation:

Clean the pair, simmer, and slice into elongated segments. Incorporate the spices into the oil and introduce a double portion. Incorporate water into the mixture and proceed with the cooking process.

Once the texture reaches a near-soft consistency, incorporate the thinly sliced onion and the precooked white beans. Allow the flame to persist until all components have reached a tender consistency.

Easy Creamy Oatmeal

Ingredients

2 tablespoons walnuts, chopped

1 cup instant oatmeal

1 banana

2 cups low-fat milk

Method

Incorporate the oatmeal and low-fat milk in a bowl that is safe for use in a microwave.

Adjust the microwave setting to high and proceed to cook the oatmeal for approximately a duration of 2 minutes.

Take out the oatmeal from the microwave oven and proceed to agitate it until it attains a creamy consistency.

Remove the peel from the banana and proceed to meticulously crush it; incorporate the thoroughly mashed banana into the bowl containing the oatmeal. Stir well until well-combined.

Garnish the oatmeal with finely chopped walnuts and promptly serve.

Berry Blast Off

- 1 c. granola, low-fat
- 1 c. low-fat yogurt, plain 1 c. washed strawberries, cut into slices
- 1 c. washed blueberries or other fruit
-

Please procure four small-sized glasses.

Distribute the strawberries evenly among the glasses.

Employ granola as a garnish atop the strawberries.

Divide the blueberries and sprinkle granola over them.

Place a dollop of yogurt onto the surface of the blueberries.

The Impact Of Weight Loss On Individuals Following The Dietary Approaches To Stop Hypertension (Dash) Regimen

Employing the DASH diet yields both positive and negative outcomes.

Individuals who adhere to the principles of the DASH Diet have demonstrated notable success in reducing their blood pressure levels. That is, after all, the primary objective that the strategy was designed to accomplish. Due to this reason, adhering to its dietary recommendations would be a prudent course of action.

Thus far, it has been recognized as the most superior approach to achieve weight loss. Shedding excess weight is inherently the most effective approach to naturally reduce elevated blood pressure levels, provided that one is suffering from obesity.

Our systolic pressure can be decreased by 5 to 20 units for every 20 pounds of excessive weight we lose. In the event of obesity, a reduction in weight by as little as 10 pounds can potentially serve to mitigate or prevent elevated blood pressure levels.

Individuals who have diabetes in conjunction with high blood pressure stand to gain an additional advantage. Individuals with diabetes have expressed that the DASH diet is highly effective in promoting a healthy eating lifestyle. Furthermore, it ranks among the top choices as an optimal dietary regimen for managing their condition.

Shedding excess weight is the most efficient approach to reduce your blood pressure and deter its recurrence. The DASH Diet has the potential to facilitate weight loss and effectively reduce blood pressure levels.

Our objective is to render the need for a physician obsolete. It is inevitable to forgo preventive care, however, we may selectively utilize their services when warranted. The occurrence of elevated blood pressure can be regarded as a consequential aspect of the aging process or the condition of being overweight. Engaging in regular physical activity and adhering to a nutritious diet can contribute to the reduction or elimination of this potential hazard.

Having a blood pressure exceeding 134/84 is known as hypertension. The DASH diet prioritizes the reduction of sodium intake as well as the maintenance of a suitable percentage of body fat during the weight loss process.

If one were to regulate their caloric intake to a degree that sustains an equilibrium of energy at a weight considered healthy, the DASH diet has the potential to facilitate weight loss and prevent the onset of obesity. This diet effectively addresses the issues of obesity and hypertension. Researchers were unable to explore the factors involved in initiating and sustaining the process.

Investigations have been undertaken to examine the motivational and introspective prerequisites of individuals striving to achieve and sustain weight loss. There are enduring advantages to acquiring knowledge and implementing these methodologies. It is possible to attain and sustain weight reduction beyond the targeted level of body fat. These skills can be refined through practice and guidance. In the majority of instances, you will encounter prevalent matters that have already been addressed in alternative sources.

Due to insufficient knowledge, inadequate time allocation, and a dearth of enthusiasm, a significant number of our medical practitioners and other healthcare providers find themselves unable or incapable of imparting aforementioned knowledge to their patients. You are henceforth solely accountable for your personal welfare.

This exceeds the capacity of many individuals. If you desire a change in circumstances, it is within your power to bring about that change. Each and every individual has the ability to effect positive change within this community.

Mixed Tomato Salad

Ingredients:

- cherry tomatoes, 1 ½ cups, orange, halves
- red cherry tomatoes, 1 ½ cups, halves
- basil, 4 leaves, chopped
- Salt and pepper to taste

- red wine vinegar, 2 tbsp.
- shallots, 1 tbsp., minced
- olive oil, 1 tbsp.
- pear tomatoes, 1 ½ cups, yellow, halves

Directions:

1. To prepare the dressing, acquire a

petite bowl. Proceed to blend together red wine vinegar, shallot, salt, and pepper, ensuring a thorough amalgamation of the ingredients.

In a spacious bowl, combine all of the tomatoes. Proceed to apply the dressing generously over the tomatoes, ensuring that each layer is adequately coated, followed by a gentle scattering of finely chopped basil.

Enjoy!

The Health Advantages And Contraindications Of The Dash Diet

The DASH diet has garnered significant attention and acclaim due to its extensive clinical research foundation. This diet has been extensively investigated, primarily due to its remarkable efficacy in reducing blood pressure and enhancing cardiovascular well-being. The aforementioned objectives were pursued during the study conducted in the 1990s, however, the diet has since progressed to offer multiple health advantages.

What are the potential health advantages associated with following the DASH diet?

Lose weight.

The DASH diet distinguishes itself from other dietary approaches by prioritizing heart health enhancement over weight reduction, as its primary goal revolves around lowering sodium and fat consumption levels. However, the empirical evidence demonstrates that adherence to the DASH diet is indeed effective in facilitating weight loss. By eliminating the consumption of detrimental carbohydrates, sugars, and fats from your dietary regimen, while concurrently increasing your incorporation of highly fibered fruits, vegetables, and lean sources of protein, it is plausible that a reduction in body mass may be observed due to the adoption of these nutritionally advantageous food selections. According to a research paper published in the esteemed Archives of Internal Medicine Research Journal, it was observed that individuals who adhered to the DASH diet while simultaneously integrating exercise into their routine experienced a significant weight loss of approximately 20 pounds. In the current context of society's emphasis on health, a significant portion of individuals are actively striving to adopt a lifestyle that incorporates increased physical activity. Incorporating physical activity into your weekly regimen, alongside the adoption of a nutritious DASH diet, can contribute to weight reduction and subsequently decrease the likelihood of developing ailments such as diabetes, obesity, and heart disease. It is a mutually beneficial situation.

Lower BP.

As previously discussed within the context of the diet's historical background, the primary objective of this dietary regimen was to address the escalating concern of hypertension by conscientiously modifying one's food choices and closely managing one's salt consumption. The DASH diet endeavors to reduce strain on the heart during the circulation of blood by maintaining a proportional consumption of unhealthy fats and sodium. This measure can serve as a preventative measure against a condition known as atherosclerosis, wherein the body's arteries constrict as a result of the heightened blood pressure. The preliminary findings of the DASH diet trial indicate that adhering to the dietary regimen for a mere two weeks can result in a reduction in blood pressure. Notably, it is worth mentioning that the DASH diet exhibits the ability to lower blood pressure levels in individuals who are both healthy and those diagnosed with hypertension.

Mitigate the development of osteoporosis and uphold bone density.

A significant portion of the food items recommended on the DASH diet offer a considerable supply of protein, potassium, vitamin D, and calcium. These nutrients serve as crucial elements in preserving bone density and retarding the progression of osteoporosis. As the aging process ensues, the inherent inclination of our physiological system is the gradual depletion of both muscular and osseous mass. This phenomenon is observed at a higher frequency among women and specific ethnic groups across the globe. Moreover, studies have indicated that a decrease in sodium consumption can have positive effects on the overall health of the skeletal system. Incorporating nutrient-rich foods such as leafy green vegetables, fruits, dairy products, and whole grains into your diet can effectively nourish your bones with a diverse range of essential nutrients, minerals, and potent antioxidants, thereby ensuring their optimal health. This can mitigate the rate of bone demineralization and maintain your physical agility and mobility for an extended period of time.

Mitigate the likelihood of developing diabetes.

Research indicates that the adoption of the Dietary Approaches to Stop Hypertension (DASH) diet has demonstrated the capacity to ameliorate insulin resistance and reduce the susceptibility to developing Type 2 diabetes. Through the exclusion of starchy foods and refined grains from one's dietary intake, the body experiences a reduction in the production of easily digestible glucose molecules, which in turn mitigates the elevation of blood sugar levels. Upon the detection of an increase in glucose levels by the body's receptors, the pancreas proceeds to secrete insulin in order to facilitate the transportation of glucose to the cells throughout the body. The issue arises when an excess of blood sugar spikes occur, overwhelming the body's capacity to sufficiently respond with insulin. This can result in an erratic level of glucose and insulin in the bloodstream, potentially resulting in the development of diabetes. By adopting the DASH diet, which emphasizes the consumption of a greater amount of fruits and vegetables and a reduced intake of carbohydrates, individuals can effectively mitigate their susceptibility to diabetes.

Improve kidney health.

Elevated sodium consumption has been shown to contribute to renal failure owing to the strain it imposes on the kidneys in expelling excessive waste and minerals from the organism. The National Kidney Foundation has endorsed the utilization of the DASH diet as a recommended dietary approach for individuals who are highly susceptible to kidney failure and seek to proactively avert the development of kidney stones. Kidney stones arise from the accumulation of minerals within the renal cortex. Certain stones possess a diminutive nature, enabling their passage through the urinary tract, while others assume a larger size which triggers pronounced discomfort. The DASH diet effectively mitigates the accumulation of surplus minerals, thereby alleviating the risk of kidney stone formation. According to scientific research, an overconsumption of sodium and an inadequate intake of calcium have been identified as factors that can elevate the risk of developing kidney stones. Fortunately, the DASH diet endeavors to diminish the amount of sodium one consumes while promoting the intake of nourishing dairy products.

Reduces the risk of developing cardiovascular conditions.

According to research conducted at the National Institute of Health, women who adhered to the DASH diet exhibited a reduction of approximately 20% in their risk levels. The primary objective of the DASH diet is to alleviate the cardiac strain resulting from the body's elevated blood pressure demands. This leads to an excessive burden on the overall cardiovascular system, potentially elevating the likelihood of experiencing a stroke or cardiac arrest. By setting a goal to lower your blood pressure, you will be supporting the well-being of your heart. Additionally, adhering to the DASH diet will result in a decrease in the consumption of detrimental fats, subsequently leading to reduced cholesterol levels. Ultimately, this will help maintain the health and integrity of your blood vessels, preventing the accumulation of plaque and other deposits. This aids in the enhancement of proper blood flow and reduces the risk of developing cardiovascular conditions.

May reduce the likelihood of developing specific forms of cancer.

According to a study carried out in 2015 at the Isfahan University of Medical Sciences in Iran, adherence to the DASH diet was associated with a reduced risk of developing various types of cancer, including breast and rectal cancer. It has been postulated by the scientific community that this phenomenon can be attributed to the notable consumption and diversity of nutrients, minerals, and dietary fiber. Fruits and vegetables that are abundant in dietary fiber have a tendency to maintain bowel regularity and enhance gastrointestinal well-being. Enhancing one's ability to eliminate surplus waste will result in improved gut and digestive system health. Moreover, vegetables and fruits possess abundant natural antioxidants that facilitate the reparative process, enhance the body's immune response, and inhibit the transformation of free radical molecules. By decreasing the consumption of detrimental fats, processed food, excessive sodium, and sugar, you are establishing a foundation for improved dietary patterns that have the potential to safeguard against specific ailments such as cancer.

It has the potential to mitigate the likelihood of depressive tendencies.

According to a study conducted in 2018 by the American Academy of Neurology, individuals who adhered to dietary patterns such as the DASH diet or those closely resembling it, such as the Mediterranean diet, demonstrated a reduced likelihood of developing depression when compared to those following alternative dietary regimens. Preliminary studies and systematic inquiries of those groups revealed a modest correlation in the findings, but further investigation would be necessary. Researchers posit that it may be attributed to the consumption of fresh fruits and vegetables rich in antioxidants. In addition, you are refraining from consuming red meat and instead focusing on incorporating lean sources of protein such as poultry and fish into your diet. Fish is abundant in omega three fatty acids, which have been scientifically demonstrated to be indispensable for brain health and the proper functioning of nerve cells.

Improve your health overall.

The DASH diet entails more than just altering your eating habits; it necessitates prioritizing your overall well-being. You are implementing several concurrent measures to modify your dietary habits, including reducing consumption of processed foods, limiting weekly sugar intake, curbing salt consumption, elevating the incorporation of vegetables, fruits, and whole grains in your diet, and actively striving to engage in more physical activity in your daily routine. By adhering to the DASH diet, one can attain these objectives pertaining to enhanced well-being, integrating all these facets of healthier living. If you are sincerely endeavoring to harness all these attributes, it is indeed possible to shed surplus pounds, despite the fact that weight loss is not the primary objective of the DASH diet. The manner in which you embrace the diet and integrate it into your everyday routine is what will prove effective for you. Adhering to a more conservative approach towards the consumption of sweets and alcohol will lead to enhanced physical well-being. If you aspire to derive benefits beyond mere blood pressure reduction, you also possess the ability to accomplish additional objectives!

Given the numerous health advantages associated with the DASH diet, it is evident why this dietary regimen has garnered considerable acclaim. While initially designed with the intention of lowering blood pressure, its manifold impacts have rendered it increasingly enticing to individuals seeking to enhance their overall well-being. By reducing your salt consumption, you can effectively mitigate the chances of developing diabetes, enhance your cardiac well-being, and promote optimal kidney function. Due to its diverse range of ingredients and straightforward instructions, it is evident why the DASH diet has garnered such popularity.

Contradictions of the DASH Diet

The DASH Diet is a common diet that is followed by millions of people in the United States. DASH is highly praised by numerous individuals, and the widely acknowledged consensus is that it represents an exceptional weight loss program. Nevertheless, the diet does come with its own drawbacks, which may become apparent upon diligent evaluation.

DASH is not widely regarded as the most optimal weight loss program within the industry. Firstly, the diet purports to facilitate weight reduction through the loss of adipose tissue. Nonetheless, there lacks substantial evidence to demonstrate its superiority over alternative weight loss methodologies. DASH displays a notably deficient level of efficacy. Additionally, certain studies assert that the DASH diet may have adverse effects on one's health.

The DASH diet permits the restricted consumption of certain food and beverage items.

When discussing the DASH diet, it is recommended to incorporate a variety of fresh fruits and vegetables into your daily consumption. It is permissible to consume them in their additive-free form. Additionally, it is imperative that you exercise careful discernment when it comes to the consumables' constituents. Excessive consumption of ingredients such as sugar, caffeine, and others may have detrimental effects on one's health. The overarching principle of the DASH diet revolves around the necessity to moderate the consumption of the aforementioned types of food.

The distinguishing feature of the DASH diet lies in its ability to suppress the actions of vigorously active microorganisms. Nevertheless, the DASH diet has the potential to pose significant risks for a considerable number of individuals. If you have diabetes, the DASH diet may not be suitable for your health needs. It is imperative to incorporate a substantial quantity of vegetables into your diet. Nevertheless, how would you be able to partake of them if they are not adequately cooked? As a result of incorporating vegetables into your diet, you will also need to take in a significant amount of sugar. Consequently, the probability of developing diabetes is significantly increased on this particular dietary regimen. Hence, it comes as no astonishment that the DASH diet has evidenced the least efficacy among weight loss regimens.

Mediterranean Diet

The Mediterranean Diet is an additional highly-rated, evidence-based dietary regimen. Similar to the DASH Diet, there are no prescribed calorie limits and no food restrictions in place. However, it is advisable to opt for nourishing food options. On the Mediterranean diet, one would consume a generous amount of fruits, vegetables, fish, nuts, seeds, legumes, and whole grains, in accordance with the recommendations provided by the United States Department of Agriculture (USDA).

Nevertheless, the Mediterranean diet advocates for the consumption of healthful plant-based oils, such as olive oil. Consequently, it is likely that you will consume a higher amount of fat while adhering to the Mediterranean diet. Nevertheless, it is probable that the fats in question consist of predominantly polyunsaturated and monounsaturated fats, which are regarded as healthier options compared to saturated fats.

Similar to the DASH diet, extensive research has been conducted on the Mediterranean diet, confirming its significant positive impact on health. This dietary approach is associated with a reduced likelihood of developing cardiovascular diseases, metabolic syndrome, certain types of cancer, obesity, and diabetes. This evidence suggests that adopting a Mediterranean diet can yield substantial health benefits.

Flexitarian Diet

The Flexitarian Diet is a dietary approach that embraces vegetarianism while incorporating a higher level of adaptability. This dietary approach has also received high accolades from health professionals due to its emphasis on plant-based consumption while allowing for occasional inclusion of meat-based meals, which can potentially enhance compliance.

Certain individuals adhering to a flexitarian diet primarily consume a vegetarian diet, occasionally incorporating meat into their meals. However, there are individuals who adhere to a dietary regimen outlined in a published guide. By adhering to the dietary guidelines outlined in the esteemed publication authored by registered dietitian Dawn Jackson Blatner, individuals can anticipate a consumption pattern characterized by meals that are consciously limited in caloric content. Your overall daily caloric consumption will amount to approximately 1,500 calories. You will partake of a diverse array of food groups, in accordance with the recommendations set forth by the United States Department of Agriculture.

A diet centered around plant-based foods additionally offers well-documented advantages for one's health, which include a decreased susceptibility to conditions such as heart disease, high blood pressure, and diabetes.

Mayo Clinic Diet

The Mayo Clinic diet is comparable to the DASH diet in the sense that it was formulated by medical professionals with the aim of enhancing aspects linked to cardiovascular well-being. Nevertheless, it distinguishes itself from the other programs mentioned in that it operates as a subscription program with associated fees. The program is affordably priced, nevertheless, and guarantees to facilitate weight reduction and enhance overall well-being.

Men may consider consuming a daily caloric intake ranging from 1,400 to 1,800 calories. Women have the option to adhere to a dietary plan consisting of 1,200 to 1,600 calories. The dietary options prescribed within this program will aid in achieving the nutritional guidelines set forth by the USDA.

Compote Of Apples And Oatmeal Bars

Ingredients:

2 cups rolled oats

1 tablespoon of baking powder

For topping:

2 tablespoons of. chopped nuts

2 tablespoons of brown sugar

1 fresh egg

1 chopped apple

½ cup of sweetened applesauce

1 ½ cups non-fat or 1% milk

¼ tablespoon of salt

1 tablespoon of cinnamon

1 tablespoon of vanilla

2 tablespoons of. oil

Directions:

To begin, it is necessary to preheat the oven to 375 degrees. Subsequently, the baking tray, measuring approximately 8" x 8", should be lightly coated with oil and set aside. At this juncture, transfer the rolled oats into a bowl and combine the cinnamon, baking powder, and salt. Blend together all of the components and set them aside. Retrieve a distinct vessel in which you may vigorously whisk the egg, and subsequently incorporate the milk, vanilla, and applesauce. Subsequently, carefully incorporate the oil and proceed to transfer the egg mixture into the mixture of rolled oats. Endeavor to thoroughly blend the ingredients once more until they are fully integrated. Next, carefully transfer this mixture into the adequately prepared baking tray before carefully placing it into the oven. Proceed to cook all ingredients for a duration of 30 minutes until uniformly golden. Take out from the oven and evenly distribute the 2 tablespoons of brown sugar on top. Reposition the item in the oven tray once more and allow it to remain for a duration of 5 minutes. Abstract from the heat source and slice into desired shapes before presenting. You may opt to store the remaining squares in the refrigerator for future utilization.

Cocoa Infused Pudding Beverage

Ingredients:

- 1 packet Splenda or stevia
- 2 tablespoons unsweetened cocoa powder
- 1 cup vanilla soymilk
- ½ medium bananas, chopped
- ¼ avocado, pitted, peeled, chopped

Directions:

1 Blitz together soymilk, bananas, avocado, Splenda, and cocoa powder in a blender until you get a smooth puree.
2 Pour into a tall glass and serve with ice, if desired.

Baked Fresh Eggs With Swiss Chard, Feta, And Basil, Cooked Sunny-Side Up.

Ingredients:

- ⅛ teaspoon of freshly ground black pepper
- 4 cups of Swiss chard, chopped
- ¼ cup of crumbled feta cheese
- 4 large fresh eggs
- ¼ cup of fresh basil, chopped or cut into ribbons
- 1 tablespoon of extra-virgin olive oil, divided
- ½ red onion, diced
- ½ teaspoon of kosher salt
- ¼ teaspoon of nutmeg

Directions:

Set the oven temperature to 375°F in advance. Position four ramekins onto a half sheet pan or within a baking dish, then lightly coat them with a thin layer of olive oil.

Proceed to warm the remaining olive oil in a generously-sized skillet or sauté pan over a moderate heat. Incorporate the onion, salt, nutmeg, and pepper, then proceed to sauté until achieving translucency, typically taking around 3 minutes. Incorporate the chard into the mixture and proceed with stirring, allowing it to wilt for approximately 2 minutes.

Distribute the mixture evenly among the four ramekins. Place 1 tablespoon of feta cheese into each individual ramekin. Place 1 egg atop the mixture in each ramekin. Place in the oven and cook for a duration of 10 to 12 minutes, or until the egg white has fully solidified.

Permit to cool for a duration of 1 to 2 minutes, subsequently proceed with caution to delicately relocate the fresh eggs from the ramekins onto a plate using a fork or spatula. Garnish with the basil.

Cooking advice: should one choose to leave the fresh eggs within the ramekins subsequent to their removal from the oven, the fresh eggs will undergo further cooking. If you desire to present the fresh eggs in the ramekins, it is advisable to remove them from the oven slightly ahead of time (around 8 to 10 minutes), in order to prevent excessive cooking of the yolks.

Guidelines For Initiating The Process

Our comprehensive 21-day regimen offers detailed instructions and justifications for the recipes we have included, along with valuable insights and strategies to assist you in seamlessly transitioning from a three-week program to a sustained modification in your lifestyle. The plan is formulated in accordance with a 2,000-calorie dietary regimen and could potentially be adjusted through the implementation of portion reduction or the modification of snack and dessert timings. By adhering to the 21-day program, you will be able to develop regular patterns and gain proficiency in organizing a week's worth of meals, regardless of whether you are preparing food for yourself or a large group. Presented herein are a selection of invaluable strategies that shall facilitate your adaptation to this transition.

Preparation is Key

The primary motivation behind dining at restaurants or consuming pre-packaged microwaveable meals is typically one of practicality. Dining at restaurants frequently serves as the backdrop for commemorating significant events or as a convenient alternative when meals at home are neither expeditiously prepared nor appetizing. Envision a scenario where you have access to superior alternatives conveniently in your culinary space. Our cookbook places significant emphasis on nutritious replacements for snacks, meals, and condiments, offering numerous options that are undoubtedly more enticing than what one would typically encounter at fast-food establishments.

The efficacy of this dietary approach resides in effectively utilizing one's weekends or evenings, wherein ample time can be allocated to meal preparation for the entire week. Having meals prepared in advance makes you less likely to eat out or reach for something less healthy. The implementation of the plan is further facilitated if all residents within your household adhere to it. It is a matter of simplicity: in the event that there is no purchase of delectable chips or cookies that lack nutritional value, one's ability to partake in said items from one's cupboard shall be rendered impossible. Even for culinary preparations of a more elaborate nature, it is feasible to conveniently slice fruits and vegetables for subsequent utilization throughout the week. As an illustration, the act of pre-dicing onions and squash eliminates a significant portion of the time required to prepare our turkey chili formula.

Ultimately, engaging in meal preparation ahead of time provides an ideal means to apportion your meals accordingly. If you frequently experience time constraints in the mornings, it may be worth contemplating the preparation of a parfait the previous evening, subsequently storing it in a mason jar or a container with an airtight seal, for easy portability. Trail mix can be readily portioned into cups and serves as a nutritious snack.

Keep it Moving!

Please contemplate the possibility of engaging in a brisk stroll or engaging in light-to-moderate physical activity as an integral component of this proposed strategy. In line with the guidelines set forth by the USDA, reducing sodium consumption is highly recommended, alongside the incorporation of regular physical activity, consisting of 30 minutes per day for 5 days each week, as a fundamental component of maintaining overall well-being. By engaging in preliminary vegetable preparation, strategically arranging meals and snacks, and preserving sauces through canning, you may discover an increase in available time throughout the workweek to engage in physical activity. Do you find yourself lacking sufficient time to engage in a 30-minute exercise routine on a daily basis? Take into account allocating a span of 10-15 minutes each day, even in situations of limited time, and compensate for it at a later point during the week. The duration of your daily workout is inconsequential, provided that you accomplish a total of 2 hours and 30 minutes of exercise per week. Ensure that you engage in a consultation with your physician to ascertain the appropriate tier of the diet for you, as well as the recommended level of physical activity.

Support your local community by purchasing products that are in season.

Engaging in seasonal shopping allows individuals to access an array of fresh produce that is abundant in essential nutrients and phytochemicals. By opting for produce that is cultivated within the local vicinity, you can actively contribute to the welfare of community vendors and farmers, enhance your understanding of the ingredients utilized in your culinary preparations, and partake in the consumption of vital nutrients that are seasonally optimal for the body.

The Fundamental Factor For Achieving Weight Loss, Weight Gain, Or Weight Maintenance With Simplicity

Regrettably, a lack of self-awareness regarding their own physiological requirements frequently renders many individuals insufficiently guided by the uncomplicated yet highly impactful fundamental principles for a wholesome dietary regimen. However, it is imperative that the subsequent regulations are established as fundamental pillars of your personal dietary regimen.

Consume a plentiful variety of fruits, vegetables, and whole, unprocessed foods.

Consume food when you experience hunger.

Consume until you have satisfied your hunger.

Consume nourishment when you sense a depletion of energy within your physical being.

Despite its apparent simplicity, this concept poses a challenge for numerous individuals when it comes to execution. For individuals who find these rules to be overly loosely defined, leaving room for ambiguity and flexibility, the subsequent straightforward steps are essential for achieving success. In a methodical manner, you will acquire the knowledge and skills necessary to accurately monitor and manage your caloric intake with ease, leading to the realization of your objectives while minimizing deprivation.

"Please be mindful of the following:

If one consumes a higher quantity of calories than one expends, weight gain will occur.

If one consumes a caloric intake that is lower than the amount expended, weight loss is experienced.

These two principles serve as the foundation for achieving success. Initially, it is essential to diligently engage in calorie counting (if you genuinely aspire to achieve optimal results); however, you will swiftly develop the ability to accurately gauge portion sizes and caloric values without the need for meticulous documentation. One quickly attains a sense of it. Due to the excessive consumption of healthful foods, weight gain may still occur. Certainly, utilizing the mirror as a reference can be helpful. However, for many individuals, particularly during the initial stages, the practice of calorie counting proves to be advantageous. Due to the presence of explicit instructions that can be complied with, you are able to gain a better understanding of food.

You will be assessed on Sunday mornings.

Maintain your regular dietary habits for a duration of one week, while diligently logging the calorie intake within a designated mobile application.

Please reassess your weight after the passing of one week.

Sum up the caloric intake over the course of the week and compute the average daily value. For example, a total of 21,000 calories per week would equate to an average intake of 3,000 calories per day.

Please perform a comparison between your weight measured at the start of the week and your weight recorded at the end.

If there has been an increase in your body weight, it is imperative that you consume a caloric intake of less than 3,000.

If you have experienced weight loss, it is recommended to maintain your current dietary pattern for an additional week to evaluate whether your weight loss persists.

Thus, it is advisable to diligently monitor your caloric intake, observe the corresponding physiological responses in your body, and accordingly modify the calorie consumption aligned with your specific objectives. If it becomes evident that weight loss is not occurring with the consumption of 2,500 calories, it is advisable to make a reduction of 200 calories and reassess the results. When making selections for the caloric intake of your meals, the same fundamental principles are applicable once more.

Aim to consume a daily quantity of fruit ranging from 200-250 grams.

Endeavor to consume 500 grams of vegetables daily.

Seek out sources of nutritious fats

Make an effort to refrain from consuming wheat and refined sugar.

Please ensure you consume ample amount of water.

Strive to obtain the majority of your caloric intake from nutritious sources, ideally ranging from 70-80%.

It is of no consequence if the remaining 20-30% of the calorie intake is derived from indulging in one's preferred confections or other nutritionally deficient substances.

A prevalent belief held by numerous individuals is that one must abstain from excessive indulgence and adhere exclusively to a nutritionally balanced diet in order to achieve effective weight loss. A balanced diet, similar to various aspects of life, remains largely unaffected when consumed in moderation. If your dietary intake comprises primarily of nutritious foods comprising at least two-thirds of your overall choices, and you adhere to the aforementioned guidelines, you may indulge in a serving of ice cream, a small portion of cake, or any other desired treat. If one harbors specific ambitions in the realm of competitive sports, it is imperative that this aspect be subjected to closer scrutiny, thereby necessitating a decrease in consumption of unhealthy food to a range spanning from 0% to 10%, contingent upon the nature of the aforementioned goal.

Develop a more thorough understanding of your physical well-being and refrain from subjecting yourself to excessive stress.

If you have consumed an excess amount of food on a certain day, you will subsequently reduce your intake slightly on another day.

If you have consumed a substantial amount of fat on one day, it is advisable to reduce your fat intake on the following day.

If you have consumed excessive food, simply engage in additional physical activity.

Would you be interested in partaking in a social gathering over the weekend where we can enjoy pizza and cocktails in the company of our friends? Consume a modest amount of food throughout the day.

It is advised to maintain a general understanding of your caloric intake and observe the changes in your body weight.

The aforementioned points can be extended indefinitely, however, the fundamental concept ought to be evident to all. Consume predominantly nutritious foods, familiarize yourself with your body, and make an assessment of caloric intake. This enables you to attain your personal weight objectives in a wholly tranquil manner, devoid of excessive strain and limitations. Exert genuine effort in commencing the task of organizing your groceries within a user-friendly mobile application. "Upon the elapse of a specific duration, the majority of commonly utilized ingredients are accumulated within the"

With the utilization of the application, there is no longer a requirement to measure or determine the weight of the items, as an estimation can now be made. It is highly likely that there will come a time when you will no longer need to input them, given that you possess a general understanding of the caloric content of your meals.

Summary:

Determine your required calorie intake

Gradually incorporate nutritious foods into your dietary regimen while progressively eliminating consumption of unhealthy foods.

Gradually acclimate oneself to the new dietary regimen and establish it as a lasting practice.

Foster an understanding of your physical well-being and cultivate an intuition regarding its requirements, such as the appropriate caloric intake for weight loss or gain, as well as the dietary choices necessary for enhanced vitality and well-being.

How to maintain a high level of motivation

During the journey towards achieving a toned abdomen and improving overall well-being, self-motivation can serve as a valuable form of assistance. The technique known as neurolinguistic programming, commonly referred to as NLP, is regarded by a certain segment of individuals as the preferred approach. NLP is primarily employed as a sales technique; nevertheless, it can also be utilized for personal motivation purposes. In order to accomplish this, it is necessary to possess some knowledge regarding the approach. Neurolinguistic programming can be defined as the process of actively modifying the neural connections associated with language. This statement refers to the restructuring of stimulus-response sequences in humans. Through the process of analyzing one's previous behavior and reprogramming it, an individual can effectively modify and alter their own conduct. Natural Language Processing (NLP) concentrates on strategies and patterns of communication to examine the process of perception. The objective of NLP revolves around communication focused on achieving success. NLP originated as a significant departure from the realm of scientific psychology. NLP is largely dismissed as lacking scientific rigor within the scholarly literature focused on psychology.

Nevertheless, individuals utilizing NLP tools are inclined towards self-motivation in transitioning from a problematic state to a desired state of achievement. Steering clear of obstacles, heading towards objectives. The news of yesterday lacks captivating appeal and provides limited value unless one derives wisdom from errors, adhering to the dictum: Each setback fortifies my resilience. By employing various NLP techniques, individuals are able to elicit and harness their internal motivations to either prevent or actively pursue specific states and behaviors. Primarily, it is essential that the work is enjoyable. In our particular situation, this implies that in order to achieve your objective of attaining a "flat stomach" or enhancing your vitality and performance, it is imperative for you to derive pleasure from the process. For instance, this could encompass promoting a superior standard of living for yourself, ensuring that you can comfortably fit into your previous pants, or simply becoming more appealing to the opposite gender. The objective you have in mind elicits a sense of optimism. Given the current circumstances, it should not be difficult for you to tap into your inner reservoir of strength and cultivate a positive and life-enhancing environment. You engage with your social milieu through effective communication, as it constitutes a vital ingredient in fostering personal self-motivation. You uphold favorable relations with your counterparts and receive constructive feedback from them, providing motivation.

You establish a socio-cultural environment that fosters the achievement of your objectives. Your future vision is appealing and coveted. You continually drive yourself by diligently ensuring the ongoing realization of your vision, consistently progressing day in and day out, week after week, and month after month. For instance, as evidenced by the gradual reduction of your waist circumference. You diligently and precisely pursue the attainment of your goals by sequentially altering your dietary habits, shedding excess body fat, engaging in rigorous physical training, and ultimately achieving the reduction of abdominal fat.

Simultaneously, you engage in an ongoing process of cognitive development, enabling you to transition from a mindset focused on problems to one focused solely on achieving objectives. Aligned with the principle of incremental progress, you can effectively tackle the objectives you have established by breaking them down into achievable increments. Please note that there will consistently be stages that are more manageable for you, as well as others that may necessitate additional effort. If complications arise despite a brief period, one can revert to the overarching objective of achieving a 'toned abdomen' or 'heightened state of wellness'.

Subsequently, direct all of your efforts towards achieving the intended advantage of the requisite subsequent actions and endeavors. Within this platform, one has the capacity to effortlessly form interconnected streams of thought. The morning ritual of taking a brief, invigorating shower in cool water can serve as illustrative evidence. Rephrase: "Reaffirm to yourself, 'If I am capable of enduring this 20-second challenge presently, it shall render my future endeavors less arduous' or 'By successfully accomplishing this task presently, it shall boost my self-assurance and consequently propel me towards achieving a greater number of my goals.'" These instances have the potential to be applied across a wide range of scenarios and can be further developed in diverse manners.

Create a motivating orientation. Subsequently, direct your attention towards the necessary incremental actions that must be taken presently. It is imperative to have a personalized approach and follow through with consistent effort. Self-motivation always stems from a compelling vision of the future. In the present circumstances, consider the hypothetical scenario of attaining a toned abdomen. What opportunities are unfolding before me? What is the level of desirability I possess? What is the expected level of value and fulfillment that my life will possess? Which medications are unnecessary for me to take? What is the increased life expectancy? What impact will this have on my overall health and well-being? Naturally, it also relies on our fundamental constitution. Do I align more with a realist perspective, an optimistic worldview, or a pessimistic outlook? Please endeavor to categorize your possessions with a high degree of realism. As a result, your thought patterns, emotional responses, and evaluative processes will inherently gravitate towards a more optimistic outlook. Strive to engage fully with the present, embracing its sensory appeal and captivating allure. Subsequently, your behavior will be influenced by an equally compelling prospective vision.

It is equally essential in the realm of NLP to indulge oneself in moments of pleasurable relaxation. Commend the achievement of intermediate objectives as triumphant milestones, alongside your companions.

Zucchini Lunch

Ingredients

- 1 cup of self-rising flour
- 1 carrot, grated
- 3 diced bacon slices
- 1 1/2 cup of cheddar cheese, grated
- 1 tsp of vegetable oil
- 3 zucchinis, grated
- 6 fresh eggs
- 1 onion, finely chopped
- Salt & black pepper

Instructions

Prior to commencing baking, adjust your oven temperature to 350 degrees Fahrenheit.

Apply a fine mist of oil onto the surface of the baking pan. Combine all of the ingredients in a bowl before transferring the mixture onto the baking pan.

Place in your preheated oven and bake for approximately 40 minutes, or until fully cooked. Ensure that it has cooled down prior to serving.

Core Principles Of The Dash (Dietary Approach To Stop Hypertension) Eating Plan

DASH stands apart from conventional diet plans due to its distinctive approach. It signifies the concept of Dietary Approaches to Prevent Hypertension. Indeed, your comprehension is accurate. At long last, we present a dietary plan that directs its attention towards one of the most significant contributors to mortality in the current era, namely hypertension. Based on recent research findings, it is evident that one in every three adults experiences hypertension or elevated blood pressure levels. It exhibits a steady incline in occurrence as individuals grow older, with almost two-thirds of the populace experiencing its effects starting from the age of 65. Elevated blood pressure is not solely associated with stroke, but rather it is linked to the development of cardiovascular complications, renal disorders, and potentially even diabetes.

The combination of our inactive lifestyles and poor dietary choices has contributed to the prevalence of numerous diseases associated with hypertension. The majority of these issues can be remedied by adhering to a nutritious diet, which aligns with the objectives of the DASH program. This dietary plan encompasses food items and culinary preparations that advocate for reduced sodium content while emphasizing elevated levels of potassium, calcium, fiber, and magnesium within the body. Additionally, it can aid in attaining ideal overall blood pressure parameters without adversely affecting physiological functions. When such an occurrence takes place, the probability of hypertensive complications decreases, including but not limited to osteoporosis, diabetes, and renal failure.

The primary objective of the initial dietary regimen was to reduce blood pressure by means of natural foods, without any reliance on medication. It received sponsorship and endorsement from the National Institute of Health in the United States. Upon the release of the initial DASH diet trials, it was established that the reduction in blood pressure effectively facilitated the maintenance of its levels, even in the presence of certain surplus amounts of sodium in the bloodstream. Furthermore, not only did the diet exhibit these effects, but it was also discovered to be advantageous in preventing weight gain. Mitigate and lower the probability of hypertension-associated ailments.

Which Individuals are Recommended to Adhere to This Dietary Plan?

Does the diet suit my needs? Alternatively, does it exclusively cater to individuals with pre-existing hypertension conditions? Based on the guidelines set forth by the Dietary

Guidelines for Americans, the DASH diet is recognized as a healthful dietary framework that is accessible to individuals of all backgrounds. Undoubtedly, individuals afflicted with hypertension are the principal recipients of the diet given its central aim of reducing blood pressure. Individuals of all ages, including children, can effectively adhere to this weight loss regimen in order to achieve improved health outcomes based on scientific principles.

This particular diet proves highly effective where other diets tend to be unsuccessful, as it ensures the body attains and maintains a sufficient intake of essential nutrients. A balanced dietary regimen promotes an increase in vital micronutrients like calcium, magnesium, and potassium, while effectively managing sodium levels. This is accomplished through an organized, systematic, and refined approach, free from any sudden fluctuations or disruptions in the body's metabolic processes, thereby promoting improved overall well-being.

The Enhanced Dietary Approaches to Stop Hypertension (DASH) Eating Plan

At the inception of hypertension-related dietary research, weight loss was not accorded excessive emphasis. Their primary focus was to ensure proper regulation of blood pressure levels. However, it was soon apparent to the researchers that prioritizing healthy weight loss became imperative, leading to the identification of an additional requirement for the development of a structured weight reduction strategy and the implementation of measures to lower blood pressure levels. Therefore, following extensive consideration, the DASH diet for weight loss was additionally developed, comprising of nuts, grains, whole fruits and vegetables, as well as seeds.

In contrast to alternative transient dietary approaches, characterized by anecdotal evidence rather than scientific backing, the DASH diet primarily draws upon scientific principles pertaining to optimal health. The investigation conducted on DASH diets suggests that it extends beyond being a mere instrument for effectively lowering blood pressure through the adoption of a low-sodium dietary approach. The plan has been meticulously crafted to cater to the individual requirements of each person, taking into account their unique needs. It encompasses a wide range of nutritious foods, including fruits, vegetables, grains, and fresh produce, that promote overall well-being and maintain optimal physical fitness. Esteemed research institutions such as the American Heart Association, Dietary Guidelines for Americans, and the National Heart, Lung, and Blood Institute have all expressed their endorsement of this dietary regimen.

Following the emergence of several additional research reports, modifications were made to enhance the DASH diet, with the goal of optimizing health and reducing hypertension. These adjustments involved augmenting protein intake while reducing the consumption of empty Carbohydrates and unhealthy fats. The fundamental proposition of the DASH diet is rooted in robust scientific principles that support achievable and enduring weight reduction. The dietary regimen includes substantial, fiber-rich foods which provide prolonged satiety and discourage impulsive snacking. They are primarily engineered to uphold stable blood sugar levels, in contrast to the fluctuating patterns observed in alternative dietary approaches. By adhering to this dietary regimen, you are able to maintain stable blood sugar levels, thereby mitigating the risk of developing conditions such as diabetes. In addition, your objective includes diminishing your triglyceride levels, eliminating excess abdominal fat, reducing LDL cholesterol, enhancing HDL levels, and attaining an overall improved state of well-being. Certainly, it is important to note that a substantial component of the dietary intake consists of protein, thereby fostering muscular development and facilitating the reduction of adipose tissue. Simultaneously, this inclination prevents the deceleration of metabolic activity, thereby facilitating the perpetuation of one's present weight.

Even if you do not have hypertension, you can still adopt the DASH diet as a means to maintain the overall health and resilience of your internal systems. During this phase of your endeavor, you will acquire knowledge on how to effectively implement this dietary regimen to suit your individual needs.

The city of Rome did not materialize overnight. Likewise, your physique will not respond favorably to abrupt alteration. It shall object, and you shall swiftly revert to the starting point. In order to alleviate such discomfort, it is advisable to proceed gradually. Consequently, it is ill-advised to hastily embark on the diet. Sample formal alternative: "Commence by implementing the meal plan for a duration of two days per week, subsequently progressing to a frequency of three times per week. Upon achieving a level of comfort and satisfaction, proceed to its permanent adoption." It is possible that you are presently consuming certain foods and snacks aligned with the DASH diet, without realizing it. Create a comprehensive inventory and ascertain which food items align with the dietary regimen's meal plan. Furthermore, please be aware that the integrity of the DASH diet does not falter when one chooses to dine outside of their home environment. There exists a plethora of alternatives and methodologies that can be employed when dining outside one's home. It is imperative to exercise caution and make wholesome selections.

Commencing the DASH dietary regimen

Now that you have been provided with the essential foundational knowledge regarding the DASH diet, let us proceed to examine its fundamental components.

This dietary plan consists of a diverse range of nutrients derived from an assortment of vegetables, fruits, dairy items, whole grains, lean meats, poultry, fish, as well as legumes such as peas and beans. Furthermore, it is enriched with minimal quantities of fat obtained from natural sources, while boasting a substantial amount of dietary fiber derived from the inclusion of sweet potatoes, cabbage, and leafy vegetables. It conforms to the established regulations of sodium and potassium content as prescribed by the United States guidelines. It is a versatile dietary regimen formulated to accommodate the requirements of diverse individuals, while diligently considering their individual culinary preferences. There exists a viable and nutritious substitute for nearly every type of culinary desire. The aforementioned is the composition of a customary DASH diet.

The Dash Diet For Managing Blood Pressure And Facilitating Weight Loss

The DASH Diet meal plan has effectively contributed to improving individuals' well-being for over two decades. Last few years, the diet is top-rated among other popular diets. The advantageous efficacy of dietary interventions in combating hypertension has already been substantiated. Allow me to provide some additional numerical evidence to strengthen our argument. Based on the findings of the National Institutes of Health, the diet has been shown to possess an efficacy rating of 3.3 out of 5 for weight loss purposes, while also demonstrating a remarkable score of 4.8 out of 5 in its ability to regulate and reduce blood pressure levels.

Elevated blood pressure can be predominantly attributed to the excessive sodium concentration within the physiological system. The salt that is commonly ingested is abundant in sodium content. The excessive accumulation of sodium results in its deposition within the walls of blood vessels. Sodium has an inherent affinity for water molecules, resulting in the initiation of water attraction and subsequent swelling and contraction of blood vessels. As a result, there is a subsequent increase in blood pressure, leading to a sensation of discomfort experienced by the individual.

Throughout the span of a 70-year existence, individuals consume an approximate quantity of sodium chloride amounting to approximately 500 kilograms. This mineral is exclusively consumed in its unadulterated state. The negative consequences associated with salt consumption should not lead to the misconception that it is inherently detrimental to our bodies. Like any other mineral, salt offers numerous advantages and plays a crucial role in maintaining the crucial water-salt equilibrium within the body, facilitating gastric juice production, and enabling oxygen transportation within blood cells. Nevertheless, an excessive consumption of it in our diet poses a precarious danger to our well-being.

The DASH diet facilitates sodium reduction in the body by imposing restrictions on and eliminating high-sodium content products from one's dietary intake. The sodium content in daily meals should not exceed 2,300 mg. Several studies have provided evidence to support the notion that reducing sodium intake to 1,500 mg can expedite the alleviation of hypertension.

Merely imposing a sodium restriction in the body will not yield the intended outcome. The diet exhibits a well-proportioned composition of essential elements responsible for maintaining optimal blood pressure levels, including potassium, magnesium, calcium, protein, and dietary fibers derived from plants. The desired outcome can only be achieved through the precise amalgamation of these substances.

The dietary regimen comprises an optimal amalgamation of diverse food categories, encompassing fruits, vegetables, grains, dairy products, meat, fish, poultry, eggs, nuts and seeds, legumes, and oils. Hence, the organism maintains equilibrium regarding the composition of numerous vital nutritional constituents.

In addition, one should also consider reducing their intake of salt, sugar, and fatty processed foods, as these contribute to elevated levels of blood cholesterol. By adhering strictly to the prescribed dietary regimen and engaging in daily physical exercise, it is conceivable to achieve a weight loss of approximately 17–19 pounds. for 4 months.

One notable benefit of the DASH diet is its moderate pace compared to many drastic approaches; an aspect that distinguishes it as a natural and appropriate dietary approach. And by adopting this dietary regimen as a long-term lifestyle choice, the shed kilograms do not regain their presence.

The Dash diet is regarded as one of the most advantageous for one's health. Whilst originally designed for individuals with hypertension, such a dietary regimen will enhance the overall well-being and vitality of all individuals.

The dash diet holds several benefits, as it comes with the endorsement of medical professionals and poses no detrimental effects on one's well-being. The DASH diet instills the practice of consuming meals in a proper manner.

Adhering to a well-balanced diet and receiving adequate healthcare are paramount. This dietary regimen aligns seamlessly with this principle, offering a nourishing and balanced meal scheme.

Top 10 Tips for DASH Diet

The Importance of Walking "The Significance of Walking "The Relevance of Walking "The Value of Walking "The

Role of Walking "The Necessity of Walking "The Vitality of Walking

Engaging in uncomplicated physical activities such as walking or cycling can effectively enhance the impact of the DASH diet, contributing to successful weight loss.

The optimal combination for achieving blood pressure stability entails engaging in at least 2 hours of walking and 30 minutes of sports activities each week. If the task appears daunting to you, it would be advisable to initiate with a 1-hour walk followed by 10 minutes of physical exercise. Gradually intensify the routine until you achieve the desired duration.

Avoid making drastic changes to your lifestyle

In order to minimize physical strain, it is recommended to gradually modify your dietary habits until they align completely with the principles of the DASH diet plan.

Develop a Nutritional Log

It will help you to realize how much food you eat per day and if it is dash diet-friendly. It is imperative to maintain regularity in adhering to such a journal. Rest assured that within a week, you will observe a notable transformation in your approach towards food.

Opt for Environmentally-Friendly Options with Every Dining Experience

Establish a regulation to incorporate green vegetables into each culinary occasion. By engaging in this activity, you will supply your body with ample fiber and potassium.

Imbibe Veganism for One Day Weekly

Constrain your intake of meat and abstain from consuming meat entirely on a weekly basis. Increase your consumption of legumes, nuts, and tofu, as they are abundant sources of dietary protein.

Fresh Box

Please prepare a snack comprising of a selection of fruits, vegetables, and rice cakes enclosed within a container. Such a container will assist you in refraining from consuming fast food that is high in sodium.

Food Labels Provide Valuable Information

It is advisable to consistently examine the nutritional information provided on food labels prior to purchasing packaged or processed food items. Through this action, you are able to more effectively regulate the sodium content.

It is important to take note that the low-sodium canned food ought to contain a sodium content of less than 140 mg per serving.

Add Spices

Spices such as rosemary, cayenne pepper, chili pepper, cilantro, dill, cinnamon, among others. has the ability to enhance the flavor and lend more delectability to non-savory dishes.

Enhance the Flavor of Your Snack

Individual preferences for snacks vary, with not all individuals demonstrating an affinity towards fruits and vegetables. For individuals of this group, the immediate transition to a dietary regimen consisting of nutritious foods can pose a formidable challenge. That is the reason why it is advisable to compile a catalogue of your preferred items and consume them throughout the day as a light refreshment. The food selection will remain suitable until you eliminate all unhealthy food from your dietary regimen.

Undergo a bi-monthly physical examination

Certain health issues cannot be rectified solely by altering one's dietary plan. The doctor's involvement in your dietary management is of utmost significance. Prior to commencing a dietary regimen, it is recommendable to undergo a comprehensive body assessment and subsequently seek regular medical consultation every two months to address any physical discomfort or health concerns. This proactive approach shall facilitate adherence to the diet while prioritizing your overall well-being.

Nutritious Pancakes Infused With Oats, Bananas, And Walnuts

Ingredients:

- 1/8 c. chopped walnuts
- ¼ c. old-fashioned oats
- 1 finely diced firm banana
- 1 c. whole wheat pancake mix

Directions:

Prepare the pancake batter according to the instructions provided on the packaging. Incorporate walnuts, oats, and diced banana. Apply a light layer of cooking spray onto the surface of the griddle. Place approximately one-quarter cup of the pancake batter onto the griddle once it is heated.

Invert the pancake when bubbles appear on the surface. Cook until golden brown. Serve immediately.

What Are The Advantages Associated With Adhering To The Dash Diet?

In addition to hypertension, a myriad of health benefits gradually emerged as experts meticulously documented the various conditions individuals acquired upon adopting the dietary regimen. Herein lies an enumeration of the widely recognized advantages that pertain to the DASH diet:

Alleviated Blood Pressure

The logical and immediate consequence of adhering to this dietary regimen is the intentional limitation of sodium consumption, thereby effectively mitigating the likelihood of developing hypertension by maintaining the viscosity of the blood at a nearly normal level. Individuals diagnosed with hypertension disorder are advised to significantly limit their consumption of sodium, while those without this medical condition should adhere to the recommended daily limit of 1500 mg.

Maintained Cholesterol Levels

Due to the emphasis on incorporating vegetables, fruits, whole grains, legumes, and nuts, the DASH eating plan facilitates adequate fiber intake, promoting the regulation of metabolic and digestive processes. Furthermore, it encourages the consumption of lean meats exclusively, while excluding saturated fats, thereby promoting the maintenance of healthy cholesterol levels in the body. It is necessary to substitute these fats with cholesterol-rich fats that promote heart health in order to ensure proper cardiovascular function.

Weight Maintenance

Enhancing weight reduction is an additional principal goal pursued by individuals adhering to the DASH eating plan. With a nourishing and hygienic dietary regimen, individuals have the capacity to shed surplus weight. Additionally, the DASH diet advocates for regular physical activity on a daily basis, which has been shown to play a crucial role in mitigating obesity. On occasion, obesity may arise from inflammation or fluid imbalances within the body, which can be effectively remedied by the progressive health approach employed by the DASH diet.

Diminished Susceptibility to Osteoporosis

Osteoporosis refers to the progressive deterioration of bone structures. Multiple factors are intertwined in this matter; its foundation lies in the depletion of calcium and vitamin D within the body. The DASH diet offers strategies and meal plans to address this insufficiency and mitigate the risk of osteoporosis, particularly among females.

Healthier Kidneys

The kidneys play a pivotal role in regulating the body's fluid balance through the orchestration of hormones and minerals. Therefore, a well-constructed dietary regimen specifically aimed at supporting renal function can effectively promote kidney health and maintain optimal functionality. The consumption of excessive amounts of salt or oxalate can lead to the formation of renal calculi. The DASH diet diminishes the likelihood of the formation of these stones within the kidneys.

Protection from Cancers

The efficacy of the Dietary Approaches to Stop Hypertension (DASH) diet in the prevention of various malignancies such as renal, pulmonary, prostatic, esophageal, rectal, and colonic cancers has been substantiated. The diet integrates all the essential components that can combat cancer and aid in the prevention of the proliferation of cancerous cells.

Prevention from Diabetes

The DASH diet has been found to be efficacious in mitigating insulin resistance, a prevalent contributor to the onset of diabetes in numerous individuals. The correlation between adherence to the DASH diet and decreased susceptibility to diabetes can be attributed to several factors, namely weight management, enhanced metabolic function, adequate hydration, regular physical activity, higher water intake, adoption of a low-sodium dietary regime, and the promotion of a healthy gut microbiome.

Improved Mental Health

One's psychological well-being is greatly influenced by the dietary choices one makes. Anxiety, depression, and insomnia are all manifestations arising from compromised physical well-being and an unhealthy way of life. The electrochemical equilibrium within the nervous system governs the entirety of neural transmission. By adhering to the DASH diet, you can establish an optimal environment to enhance cerebral function effectively.

Reduced likelihood of cardiovascular complications

The DASH diet, being specifically formulated to regulate blood pressure fluctuations, effectively safeguards the heart against the detrimental consequences of elevated blood pressure and proactively mitigates the risk of various diseases. Prolonged hypertension places strain on the cardiovascular system, leading to the deterioration of cardiac structures including the myocardium and valvular apparatus. The DASH diet serves as an effective means of mitigating these risks.

The Efficacy of the DASH Diet: A Comprehensive Evaluation

The significance of the DASH Diet was examined in initial research conducted by the National Institute of Health in the United States. Scientists were cognizant of the ramifications of such a dietary pattern; however, substantiating their assertion required empirical evidence. Consequently, three distinct dietary regimes were formulated in order to assess their respective effects. The strategy characterized by a substantial inclusion of fruits, vegetables, legumes, and non-fat dairy products emerged as the most efficacious in reducing the diastolic and systolic blood pressures by 3 mmHg and 6 mmHg, correspondingly. Although the DASH diet imposes restrictions on specific food items, it also advocates for monitoring caloric consumption. It ensures that the daily caloric consumption falls within the range of 1600 to 3100. This fact bears greater significance particularly in the context of grappling with obesity. In contradiction to the Optimal Macronutrient Intake Trial aimed at promoting heart health, the DASH diet has demonstrated remarkable achievement in diminishing habitual fat consumption and averting various cardiovascular ailments.

It presents a solution with a long-term perspective.

Individuals with hypertension cannot consistently rely on medications to maintain their long-term health stability. Irrespective of the potency of medications, they inevitably entail adverse reactions. Implementing modifications to one's dietary habits and daily routine can lead to sustainable remediation, in addition to imperative preventative measures. Hypertension is a chronic condition, and individuals diagnosed with it will indefinitely experience its impact. It is not a question of a few days; it pertains to the remainder of their lifetime. This is precisely the reason why solely employing dietary intervention can effectively mitigate high blood pressure and its related complications.

Facilitates the management of Type 2 Diabetes

In order to comprehend the correlation between the DASH diet and diabetes, it becomes imperative to delve into the fundamental factors contributing to the onset of Type 2 Diabetes. Consumption of food rich in calories or the accumulation of excess body weight both contribute to the development of insulin resistance in the body. Once you eliminate both of these factors, managing Type 2 Diabetes becomes more manageable. The DASH diet effectively addresses and regulates both these factors. To begin with, by means of its regulated method of provision and subsequently, by mitigating the prevalence of obesity. It enhances the body's insulin sensitivity, thereby mitigating the potential hazards associated with elevated blood sugar levels. Furthermore, the DASH diet establishes a benchmark for carbohydrate intake by promoting dietary equilibrium. Consequently, by limiting excessive carbohydrates, the body is able to effectively regulate its insulin production and corresponding physiological processes.

Ten Compelling Reasons Why the DASH Diet Efficaciously Yields Results

When discussing the practical implementation of the DASH diet, one can observe a greater demonstration of its efficacy as a dietary approach. In addition to an abundance of research and experiments, the underlying motivations driving individuals to explore this diet are its distinct characteristics. It fosters a sense of comfort and convenience, instilling a higher level of user compliance with its established rules and guidelines. "Below are several compelling factors that contribute to the exceptional effectiveness of the DASH Diet:

1. Easy to Adopt

The extensive array of choices encompassed by the DASH diet classification enhances its overall adaptability for individuals across the board. This is the underlying cause behind individuals finding it more convenient to transition to and leverage its genuine health advantages. It facilitates greater ease of adaptability for its users.

2. Promotes Exercise

It exhibits superior efficacy compared to other factors due to its comprehensive approach, encompassing not only dietary considerations, but also emphasizing the importance of regular exercise and consistent physical activities. This is the rationale behind its ability to generate expeditious and discernible outcomes.

3. All-Inclusive

With certain limitations taken into account, this Diet has incorporated every food item into its repertoire with specific alterations. It effectively provides us with information on the recommended and discouraged uses of various ingredients, ensuring that we avoid consuming those detrimental to our physical well-being.

4. A Methodology Encompassing Equilibrium

One of the major benefits it offers is the capacity to preserve equilibrium in our dietary habits, daily regimen, the amount of calories consumed, and the adequacy of our nutrient intake.

5. Good Caloric Check

Each meal on the DASH diet is meticulously calculated in terms of caloric content. We can effortlessly monitor the daily caloric consumption and consequently impose limitations by eliminating certain food items.

6. Prohibits Bad Food

The DASH diet recommends incorporating a greater quantity of organic and fresh ingredients into one's meals while discouraging the consumption of processed foods and unhealthy items commonly found in stores. Therefore, it fosters improved dietary practices amongst the individuals.

7. Focused on Prevention

While its efficacy in treating various ailments has been established, it is largely regarded as a preventative measure.

8. Gradual but Continuing Transformations.

The dietary plan is moderately flexible and allows for gradual adjustments in order to work towards attaining the optimal state of well-being. You have the flexibility to establish your targets on a daily, weekly, or monthly basis according to your preferences.

9. Long Term Effects

The outcomes yielded by the DASH diet are not only extraordinary, but they also endure over an extended period of time. The progress is deemed to be slow, yet its effects have a longer duration.

10. Accelerates Metabolism

The DASH diet's health-conscious principles have the capacity to stimulate and enhance our metabolism, thereby optimizing bodily functioning.